GOUT FREE

Beat Gout with Diet and Lifestyle
Changes and Live Life Gout Free!

Karl A. Minner

Also by Karl Minner:

Thought to Kindle

The Straight Talk Guide to Lawsuit Funding

Kindle Marketing Tips

Like Karl Minner on Facebook

https://www.facebook.com/pages/Karl-A-Minner/111508295849131

Connect with Karl on LinkedIn

https://www.linkedin.com/pub/karl-minner/6/360/b28

All Feedback Welcomed at:

karlminner@ymail.com

Acknowledgement:

Getting a book written, proofed and published is no small job. I want to thank the many people that were instrumental in bringing this idea to life. In particular, I would like to thank friends and family for helping me with the selection, editing and proofreading of this book.

To those who have needlessly suffered from GOUT. Better, healthier, gout free days are ahead.

Preface

Gout Free: Beat Gout with Diet and Lifestyle Changes and Live Life Gout Free!, was written for those who are currently suffering from Gout as an easy-to-use tool for understanding and beating Gout. It is intended to be of value to those who suffer from gout and for those who don't have it who would like a better understanding of it.

Its concise and practical approach is meant to provide a framework for understanding just what Gout is all about.

In recent years, there's been an explosion of gout. Simply put, the more obese we become as a nation, the more instances of gout and it crippling effects. Arguably, this rise is being driven by our increasing sedentary lifestyles coupled with our intake of processed food.

That said, roughly, this book is organized into three parts. Chapters 1-3 concern themselves with background information about Gout. Chapters 4-6 discuss treatment options. In the last part, Chapter 7, I offer some of my favorite gout friendly recipes and then in Chapter 8 the book comes to a close.

Table of Contents

Introduction

As a person who has Gout, I can safely say that it is no laughing matter. In fact, doctors say that next to childbirth and kidney stones, a gout attack is one of the most painful things a person can experience.

The "disease of kings" has now reached the masses. In the last half century alone, the condition has more than doubled. Along with obesity and hypertension, rates have steadily climbed. It now affects more than 8 million American adults and the numbers keep climbing. What is the culprit? Is it the fact that we are too sedentary and our food has become too processed?

In people who don't suffer from gout, eating purine rich foods such as red meat and shellfish can raise uric acid levels but their kidneys are efficient at eliminating it from the body in urine. However, people with gout actually have a defective mechanism for eliminating uric acid from the body – and this is thought to be a genetic predisposition.

Gout is a form of arthritis caused by high concentration of uric acid in the blood. This leads to the formation of tiny needle like crystals in the joints and kidneys (where they form kidney stones) and less commonly in other parts of the body including the spinal cord and the vocal chords. Gout is as painful as rheumatoid arthritis.

In any event, left untreated or uncontrolled, gout can form chalky lumps called tophi, which can severely damage joints, making walking and using the hands extremely painful. In extreme cases, joint replacements and even amputation is necessary.

Why I Wrote This Book?

In my case there were two motivating factors— my own struggle with poly-articular gout and my desire for people to understand it and 'beat it'.

Chapter 1: Some Gout Sufferers and Their Stories

<u>Meet Jack</u>

Jack was 33 and living life to the fullest when he had his first attack of gout. Over 20 years later, he eats, drinks and exercises and, thanks to effective medication, keeps his gout under control. He explained:

I was a 33-year-old construction worker in Fort Lauderdale when I experienced my first attack of gout. I woke suddenly in the night to an unbearable pain, as if someone had stamped on the ball of my foot. An area of my foot was shining red, and was very sensitive and inflamed. I was amazed. I didn't know what it was.

I think the hot weather triggered the attack. I was drinking too much beer and basically dehydrated. I am a very active person and would motor-cross a lot with my friends, not drinking enough water, and then go to lots of parties afterwards.

When I went to the hospital, the nurse looked at my foot and told me that I had gout. I was prescribed a medication called colchicine, which helps clear the uric acid (urate) from your blood.

Three years later, I got my second attack. Again, I was drinking too much, overeating and getting dehydrated, and I was stressed. The urate levels in my blood were very high, it felt like my blood was congealing. As the years went by, I had attacks every two weeks.

I was still taking colchicine, but it gave me diarrhea if I took too much. I would take the medication during the attacks, which would subside after three to five very painful days. During that time, I'd be lying down, unable to walk. It was very depressing.

In February 2007, I was walking along a street in Manhattan and my foot suddenly seized up. I tripped over the pavement and nearly fell under a bus. That's when I thought, something's seriously wrong here.

The doctors told me that urate crystals had accumulated in my blood that a hard white lump called a tophus had formed under the skin on my foot. A surgeon removed it and the other white residue in the joints of my big toe. He said it was one of the worst cases of gout he'd ever seen.

I started taking a drug called allopurinol, which reduces urate in the blood and helps prevent further attacks. I hadn't taken it before as it tended to trigger attacks, but I now take two tablets a day. It has controlled the gout and I feel great. My joints don't creak any more.

I've lost weight and my quality of life is great. I can do everything I used to do, although I have to avoid extreme exercise as this produces a lot of metabolites (breakdown products) in my blood, which can trigger an attack.

I still get gout occasionally, but it's just a quick attack that finishes within one day. Keeping hydrated is the key. I drink a pint of water every morning before I leave my bedroom. I also eat more sensibly and avoid foods like organ meats and certain types of fish, which increase my blood urate levels.

*****

Meet Patrick

Patrick, a business analyst, was only 24 when he started to experience episodes with the gout. He described:

I am now 49 years old and my story starts more than twenty five years ago. At twenty three years of age, I had episodes of going to bed at night and feeling a kind a dull ache in my foot. Waking up the next morning I was not able to move out of bed or even walk and the pain was the worse I had ever experienced in my life.

After this happened two or three times I went to the Doctor. He examined my foot, pulling it from side to side. No break and then a blood sample was taken. A week later, the word gout was mentioned at least I was diagnosed.

I was put on allopurinol, at this point I had the worst attack ever. I was not really told that this might happen. Unfortunately, every side effect you could have with allopurinol I got. I was taken off the drug.

I was then on the merry go round of many other drugs and learning to live with up to 6-10 attacks a year. Missing work and holidays as I was not able to travel. I call them attacks as it really did feel that I was being attacked by my own body.

Losing weight, drinking lots of water, avoiding alcohol and foods high in protein made no difference. I will have to admit that at one point I was very down and emotional. I seemed to live on diclofenac and, when needed, higher doses of pain killers.

Fifteen years ago in desperation I was put back on allopurinol at a lower dose and this time -- no side effects. Though the attacks still come up to 10 a year, I wouldn't give in and I started using a walking stick to walk. This was only possible with taking anti-inflammatories and pain killers. I could just about function but it was a fairly difficult time. There is only so much sticking your legs up in the air you can do!!

I was lucky to be given some advice by a fellow sufferer. I wish to share this as it has changed my life completely. Ten years ago I started to take a supplement called turmeric (an Indian spice), that I buy from a certain well know herbal shop found on many high streets.

I take two tablets each night before I go to bed and for me the attacks have all but disappeared. I don't know why it works it just does. I still get a sore foot for a day or so, but no anti-inflammatories or pain killers are needed.

In the last 3 years I have had only one semi bad attack and it is 10% of the pain I use to go through. I really wanted to share this as unless you suffer from gout you cannot really understand the pain.

The pain I suffered was both physical and mental as there were times when I use to think I can't go on. But I did as you learn to live with it.

I hope that some of you that suffer from gout try this remedy and that is all that it is. I hope that it works for you as well as it did for me.

*****

Meet Michael

Michael who is on Disability due to his gout was only 17 when his ordeal with gout started. He observed:

My life with gout started earlier than what most claim to be the general age of 35 and over. It is hereditary.

I started having problems at around the age of 17, thinking that whenever I had pain in my feet it was just because I was over active and maybe either sprained had a sprained ankle or stubbed my toe. After about 2 years of these Pains, my Doctor checked me for what is known as "GOUT", I asked him what it was he explained "It is the old Richman's disease" caused by too much drinking and rich diet.

4

He even said you're too young to have gout but we will test anyways. The test came back positive. That was in 1987. Attacks happened to me maybe 1 or 2 times in a year since then. Since that time my attacks have been getting worse and to the point of having severe attacks lasting upwards of 6 weeks with minor breaks in between.

Over the years I have had to rely on Ontario Social Services in between Jobs. I am by myself and have no one to ask for help. Workers that I have worked with have said that I was faking these gout attacks and would threaten to kick me off the system saying GOUT is not a disability. It is hard to work when you have attacks that would last a few weeks to even months and the employer would let me go saying your faking it.

There is a lack of public knowledge when it comes to gout, some people say Gout is not a disease, but I say why not live in my shoes for 1 year with this problem or even just 1 attack, then you might understand. Some attacks are minor some are far more severe.

As of April 1st 1999, I was finally awarded Disability for my Attacks with gout.

In 2008, my case worsened and I ended up having to have my knees replaced. I also had several noticeable Tophi on my toes, feet, knees that where large and a huge lump of tophi in my right elbow that was the size of a golf ball almost.

I am still on the road to recovery and now taking colchicine and allopurinol together. I have good days and I have bad days but at least I am not in a wheelchair as I was the last 3 years.

******

Unfortunately, gout and its crippling grip still exist across the globe. As evidenced above, you can see that gout strikes people very differently. Some have it, but never have symptoms. Some get it mildly, while others can need wheelchairs.

That said, the purpose of this book is to educate gout sufferers and non-gout sufferers alike with the aim of prevention and/or minimizing gout and its excruciating and debilitating attacks.

Chapter 2: What is Gout?

Gout is a rheumatic condition that manifests itself through recurrent attacks of acute inflammatory arthritis—a red, tender, hot, swollen joint. Although gout can occur in any joint of your body and in multiple joints simultaneously, the joint at the base of the big toe, the metatarsal-phalangeal joint, is where it typically strikes.

Gout occurs when too much of a substance called uric acid builds up in the blood; this condition is also called hyperuricemia- elevated levels of uric acid in the blood. Uric acid can come from the breakdown of old cells and from certain foods and drinks. If too much uric acid is produced, or if it isn't properly excreted, it can form tiny crystals that are deposited in joints, tendons, and surrounding tissues. For this reason, gout is called a "crystal deposit disease." It may also present as tophi, kidney stones, or urate nephropathy – a kidney disease.

Essentially it is a breakdown of the metabolic process that controls the amount of uric acid in your blood. The stiffness and swelling are a result of excess uric acid forming crystals in your joints, and the pain associated with this disease is caused by your body's inflammatory response to the crystals.

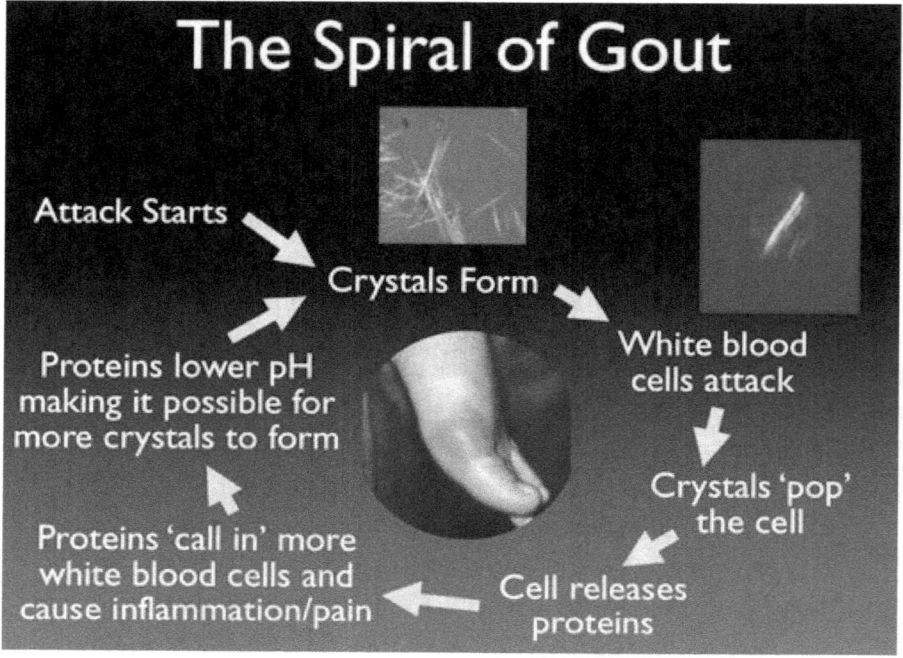

What Are the Symptoms of Gout?

A gout attack, or "flare", usually strikes suddenly, and generally at night. Mysteriously, it often targets the large joint of your big toe. Your skin becomes red, inflamed, and overly sensitive. Even the light pressure of a bed sheet can become unbearable. A fever may also be present.

The pain associated with gout is often sudden and intense. Joints tend to swell, and can be warm to the touch. The skin around the joint may also take on a deep red or purple hue. People who have had gout for extended periods of time may develop nodules beneath the skin near joints; these are accumulations of uric acid crystals. Attacks can recur in the same joint over weeks, months or years, and repeated bouts of gout can damage the joint. Kidney damage can also occur.

With or without treatment, gout symptoms will usually go away within three to 10 days, and the next attack may not occur for months, or even years, if at all. Nonetheless, if more attacks occur, they tend to increase in frequency, become more severe, and last longer. Overtime, recurrent gout attacks can damage your joints and the surrounding areas.

This is why it's important to treat your gout as soon as possible, before it begins damaging your body permanently.

What Are the Causes of Gout?

Gout has a strong genetic component. The hallmark of gout is elevated blood levels of uric acid, a breakdown product of protein metabolism (a distinction should be made by a physician between true gout and pseudo gout, a similarly painful, arthritic condition that occurs when calcium pyrophosphate dehydrate crystals are deposited in a joint). Uric acid comes from the metabolism of purines, a subclass of proteins that are abundant in human tissues and such foods as organ meats, sardines, anchovies, mushrooms, asparagus and lentils.

Moreover, a number of drugs and supplements can increase uric acid levels in the blood and its tendency to form irritating crystals in joints. These include salicylates (the active component of aspirin), vitamin B3 (niacin), excess vitamin C and diuretics that may be prescribed for high blood pressure, edema or, cardiovascular disease. Others are Cyclosporine (used to prevent rejection of transplanted organs) and Levodopa for Parkinson's disease.

Excess alcohol consumption, being overweight, and exposure to lead in the environment also increase the risk of gout in genetically susceptible individuals. Other risk factors include dehydration and acid conditions of the blood that can result from serious infections, surgery or ketogenic weight loss diets (such as the Atkins diet). The genetic component should not be underestimated, however. It is possible to have high levels of uric acid and never develop gout.

Just How Common Is Gout?

The "disease of kings" has now reached the masses. In the past half century the prevalence of gout in the general U.S. population has more than doubled. Once thought of only for the privileged few who had the means to overindulge in food and drink, gout now afflicts more than eight million American adults. And research suggests that the rates of this form of localized arthritis are still on the rise.

A new study found that some 3.9 percent of U.S. adults have been diagnosed with gout at some point. Some people have only one or infrequent flare-ups. But others are plagued by chronic, recurring symptoms. And the condition continues to affect men more often than women (some 5.9 percent of men versus 2 percent of women), according to the new analysis, which was published online July 28 in Arthritis & Rheumatism. The researchers also found that, in their study of more than 5,000 people, about 21.4 percent had high levels of uric acid in their blood, which is known to be a risk factor for developing gout.

Much of the evidence points to a link between gout and the increasing prevalence of obesity and hypertension. And as body mass indexes continue to rise worldwide, it is only going to grow.

Chapter 3: Gout Diagnosis: The Importance of Getting It Right

Many types of inflammatory arthritis, including gout, produce hot, stiff, inflamed, and painful joints. But just because someone has these symptoms doesn't necessarily mean that it's gout.

It is vital that a patient gets a proper diagnosis as Gout is a chronic disease and can lead to long-term damage.

Gout Diagnosis: Looking for Crystals

The first thing that doctors use to make an accurate diagnosis is a patient's history. Your age, sex, family history, weight, and diet are all risk factors for gout. Kidney and cardiovascular problems, as well as medications taken for these and other conditions, can also be associated with gout.

The true determinant, however, comes with a test to look for the hallmark sign of gout: uric acid crystals.

Visiting your doctor during an attack can ensure an accurate diagnosis. Drawing joint fluid during an acute attack so you can identify the uric acid crystals. The fluid is examined under a microscope with special filters so the crystals, if there are any, show up.

Bear in mind that even if crystals aren't seen in the fluid, gout can't be ruled out just yet. Further samples may be taken to see if there are crystals in the joints themselves, both those that are inflamed and others that don't appear affected. If tophi (harder, more permanent uric acid deposits) have developed, these can also be used to find uric acid, or urate crystals.

Taking fluid from swollen joints can rule out other problems, including inflammation due to infection and swelling caused by different types of crystals, such as those found in the very similar pseudo gout.

Gout Diagnosis: Looking for Hyperuricemia

Why can't a simple blood be used to diagnose gout? While most people will have elevated uric acid levels at some point during their disease, during a gout attack it's not unusual for those levels to be normal. Furthermore, levels of uric acid may also be checked in a urine sample.

However, you may not develop gout just because you have hyperuricemia. On the other hand, because people with chronic gout often have hyperuricemia when they don't have acute inflammation, blood tests may be used to monitor whether a medication is doing its job at bringing down uric acid levels.

Gout Diagnosis: Other Signs of Gout

Patients may have other physical signs of gout that last beyond the acute period. In addition to the tophi, which may develop underneath the skin — especially on the elbows and behind the ears, — uric acid may also cause kidney stones.

If tophi and perhaps kidney stones have developed, they indicate that gout has been present for a number of years, and the damage may be visible on an X-ray. The longer you go without treatment, the more likely you are to have permanent joint, and even kidney, damage. If you have hot, throbbing, almost unbearable pain in the big toe, contact your doctor. Even if the pain eases in a day or so, gout may be to blame.

In summary , the following tests to help diagnose gout may include:

- **Joint fluid test.** Your doctor may use a needle to draw fluid from your affected joint. When examined under the microscope, your joint fluid may reveal urate crystals.

- **Blood test.** Your doctor may recommend a blood test to measure the levels of uric acid and creatinine in your blood.

Remember, blood test results can be misleading, though. Some people have high uric acid levels, but never experience gout. And some people have signs and symptoms of gout, but don't have unusual levels of uric acid in their blood.

- **X-ray imaging.** Joint X-rays can be helpful to rule out other causes of joint inflammation.

- **Ultrasound.** Musculoskeletal ultrasound can detect urate crystals in a joint or in a tophus. This technique is more widely used in Europe than in the United States.

- **Dual energy CT scan.** This type of imaging can detect the presence of urate crystals in a joint, even when it is not acutely inflamed. This test is not used routinely in clinical practice due to the expense and is not widely available.

Chapter 4: What is the Conventional Treatment of Gout?

There is no known cure for gout, but it can be alleviated through a variety of conventional therapies and gout treatments. Physicians often prescribe non-steroidal anti-inflammatory drugs (NSAIDs) such as ibuprofen to keep inflammation and pain under control. Corticosteriods can have a similar affect; these are administered via pills or injections. There are also medicines that can lower levels of uric acid, the best known is probably allopurinol (Zyloprim). All of these measures should be used only as a last resort, as all carry the risk of significant side effects.

Medications to Treat Gout Attacks

Drugs used to treat acute attacks and prevent future attacks include:

- **Nonsteroidal anti-inflammatory drugs (NSAIDs).** NSAIDs include over-the-counter options such as ibuprofen (Advil, Motrin IB, others) and naproxen sodium (Aleve, others), as well as more-powerful prescription NSAIDs such as indomethacin (Indocin) or celecoxib (Celebrex).

Your doctor may prescribe a higher dose to stop an acute attack, followed by a lower daily dose to prevent future attacks.

NSAIDs carry risks of stomach pain, bleeding and ulcers.

- **Colchicine.** Your doctor may recommend colchicine (Colcrys, Mitigare), a type of pain reliever that effectively reduces gout pain. The drug's effectiveness is offset in most cases, however, by intolerable side effects, such as nausea, vomiting and diarrhea.

After an acute gout attack resolves, your doctor may prescribe a low daily dose of colchicine to prevent future attacks.

- **Corticosteroids.** Corticosteroid medications, such as the drug prednisone, may control gout inflammation and pain. Corticosteroids may be administered in pill form, or they can be injected into your joint.

Corticosteroids are generally reserved for people who can't take either NSAIDs or colchicine. Side effects of corticosteroids may include mood changes, increased blood sugar levels and elevated blood pressure.

Medications to Prevent Gout Complications

If you experience several gout attacks each year or if your gout attacks are less frequent but particularly painful, your doctor may recommend medication to reduce your risk of gout-related complications.

Options include:

- **Medications that block uric acid production.** Drugs called xanthine oxidase inhibitors, including allopurinol (Aloprim, Lopurin, Zyloprim) and febuxostat (Uloric), limit the amount of uric acid your body makes. This may lower your blood's uric acid level and reduce your risk of gout.

Side effects of allopurinol include a rash and low blood counts. Febuxostat side effects include rash, nausea and reduced liver function.

- **Medication that improves uric acid removal.** Probenecid (Probalan) improves your kidneys' ability to remove uric acid from your body. This may lower your uric acid levels and reduce your risk of gout, but the level of uric acid in your urine is increased. Side effects include a rash, stomach pain and kidney stones.

Chapter 5: Lifestyle and Diet Changes

Medications are the most proven, effective way to treat gout symptoms. However, making certain diet and lifestyle changes also may help, such as:

- Limiting alcoholic beverages and drinks sweetened with fruit sugar (fructose). Instead, drink plenty of nonalcoholic beverages, especially water.

- Limit intake of foods high in purines, such as red meat, organ meats and seafood.

- Exercising regularly and losing weight. Keeping your body at a healthy weight reduces your risk of gout.

High-Fructose Corn Syrup (HFCS)

Although gout is commonly blamed on eating too many high-purine foods, such as organ meats, anchovies, herring, asparagus and mushrooms, there is another clear culprit— high-fructose corn syrup.

Countless health problems have been linked to the consumption of high fructose corn syrup, not the least of which is gout. A recent study showed that consumption of sugar-sweetened soft drinks is strongly associated with an increased risk of developing gout.

The study, done by U.S. and Canadian researchers, indicated that men who drank two or more sugary soft drinks a day had an 85 percent higher risk of gout than those who drank less than one a month. In fact, the risk significantly increased among men who drank five to six servings of sugary soft drinks a week. Fruit juice and fructose-rich fruits, such as oranges and apples, also increased the risk

This makes sense on many levels, but first and foremost because fructose is known to inhibit the excretion of uric acid. Fructose also reduces the affinity of insulin for its receptor, which is the principle characteristic of type 2 diabetes. Furthermore, High Fructose Corn Syrup has been implicated in elevated blood cholesterol levels, and it has been found to inhibit the action of white blood cells in your immune system.

Many of the health conditions that HFCS causes, including high cholesterol and diabetes, also increase your risk of developing gout. Additionally, fructose converts more readily to fat than other sugars, making it a major risk factor for both diabetes and obesity -- another gout risk factor.

In a fructose metabolism study, it was noted that when two high-fructose breakfast drinks were consumed, the build-up of stored fat continued into the afternoon, during which time the quick conversion of fructose to fat remained active during digestion of the lunch meal. The study concluded that the higher the concentration of fructose in the diet, the higher the rate of fat conversion.

Frequently, fruit juices also have fructose added to them, and if you still believe that this is an acceptable form of sugar, think again. Fructose contains no beneficial enzymes, vitamins, minerals, or additional micronutrients. Instead, it actually leeches them from your body. Unbound fructose, found in large quantities in high fructose corn syrup, can also interfere with your heart's use of vital minerals such as magnesium, copper, and chromium.

Look At the Labels

You may think that avoiding fructose means just staying stay away from desserts and sweet drinks, but unfortunately there is more to it as fructose is hidden in many foods you would not even suspect. Names such as:: 'chicory,' 'inulin,' 'iso glucose,' 'glucose-fructose syrup,' 'dahlia syrup,' 'tapioca syrup,' 'glucose syrup,' 'corn syrup,' 'crystalline fructose,' and flat-out fraud 'fruit fructose,' or... 'agave'. Even processed meats and other foods you would never imagine contain high fructose corn syrup.

Limiting Alcohol is Crucial for Successful Gout Treatment

Gout is often seen in association with hypertension, excessive alcohol consumption, and coronary artery disease, so alcohol is a strong risk factor for this disease. In general, I believe alcohol should be reserved for people who have already achieved optimal wellness and therefore have their carbohydrates (sugars and grains) under control, and do not have disease conditions such as gout, diabetes, or other signs of ill health.

Although wine has been shown to have some health benefits, it may also increase your insulin levels, which is not only a risk factor for diabetes, but increased insulin levels have been linked with a shorter life span, in general. So it needs to be used cautiously, especially if you have gout. Most importantly for those suffering with gout, alcohol may raise the levels of uric acid in your blood, and therefore could even initiate a gout attack, so it's wise to limit the alcohol you drink, or eliminate it altogether.

Drink Water

Drink plenty of water to help flush the system. Dehydration is a major culprit of gout. To counter dehydration and minimize uric acid deposits in the joints drink 8, 8 oz glasses of water per day.

Exercise Can Dramatically Help

While exercise is not recommended while your joints are in pain or when it might cause further injury, once your gout is under control, exercise is needed as a necessary adjunct to a healthier lifestyle. Exercise will even help prevent further attacks by increasing circulation and normalizing your uric acids levels, which it does primarily by normalizing your insulin levels.

An exercise routine has other advantages as well. Studies have shown that it works as an effective antidepressant, strengthens your immune system so it can fight off diseases like cancer, and it can even improve insulin resistance and reverse pre-diabetic conditions.

Maintaining Ideal Body Weight is a Large Part of the Solution

It seems to me, one of the greatest risk factors for gout is obesity, or any excessive weight gain. Approximately half of all gout sufferers are overweight. Excess weight worsens gout because irritated nerve endings are further irritated by having to support and deal with extra weight. Furthermore, medical data shows a remarkably high prevalence of metabolic syndrome (heart disease and diabetes symptoms such as insulin resistance, abdominal obesity, hypertension, and high triglyceride levels) in gout sufferers.

Weight loss represents a safe method for reducing inflammatory states. Remember,gout is an inflammatory condition, and it is clear that losing weight, and keeping it off, will greatly improve your chances of avoiding further gout attacks.

Chapter 6: Homeopathic / Home Remedies

If gout treatments aren't working as well as you'd hoped, you may be interested in trying an alternative approach. Before trying such a treatment on your own, talk with your doctor — to weigh the benefits and risks and learn whether the treatment might interfere with your gout medication. Because there isn't a lot of research on alternative therapies for gout, in some cases the risks aren't known.

Certain foods have been studied for their potential to lower uric acid levels, including:

- **Coffee.** Studies have found an association between coffee drinking — both regular and decaffeinated coffee — and lower uric acid levels, though no study has demonstrated how or why coffee may have such an effect.

The available evidence isn't enough to encourage noncoffee drinkers to start, but it may give researchers clues to new ways of treating gout in the future.

- **Vitamin C.** Supplements containing vitamin C may reduce the levels of uric acid in your blood. However, no studies have demonstrated that vitamin C affects the frequency or severity of gout attacks.

Talk to your doctor about what a reasonable dose of vitamin C may be. And don't forget that you can increase your vitamin C intake by eating more vegetables and fruits, especially oranges.

- **Cherries.** Cherries have been associated with lower levels of uric acid in studies, as well as a reduced number of gout attacks. Eating more cherries and drinking cherry extract may be a safe way to supplement your gout treatment, but discuss it with your doctor first.

- **Apple cider vinegar**. Helping to make the body more alkaline, apple cider vinegar has become a well-known proven solution for countless ailments, including gout. Try mixing 1-2 tablespoons of apple cider vinegar in 8 ounces of water. You can either drink it in one sitting or sip on it over time – try both methods and see which is more effective. This solution can reduce pain by 90% within a day or two.

- **Baking Soda**. Among other home remedies for gout is the use of baking soda. Mixing baking soda in water can effectively relieve pain almost instantly, though it may take 1-2 days. Mix 1/2 teaspoon baking soda in 8 oz. of water and drink it in one sitting. You may need to repeat this a few times a day, taking as much as 3 teaspoons total. Reduce the dose as the pain goes away. Note: The maximum recommended dose is 4 teaspoons throughout the day. Lastly, use caution if you suffer from hypertension, as baking soda may raise blood pressure when taken in larger amounts.

- **Bromelain/ Pineapples.** a compound that can be found in pineapples or in a supplement form. The enzymes within are frequently recommended for people with gout and have even been shown to have anti-cancer properties.

- **Beet juice.** Beet juice can help prevent acidosis and stimulates the liver to cleanse bile ducts.

- **Turmeric.** Turmeric has been gaining popularity in the last few years as a home remedy for gout. Use it to reduce inflammation and oxidative stress.

Chapter 7: My Favorite Gout Busting Recipes

Gout shouldn't keep you from enjoying your food. Stick to low-purine fare, like that in the following recipes, to have a tasty meal without triggering an attack or making a flare-up worse.

1.

Sage and Garlic Grilled Chicken Breasts

Ingredients:

- 1 teaspoon dried sage leaves
- ½ teaspoon seasoned salt
- ½ teaspoon dried marjoram leaves
- ¼ teaspoon coarse ground black pepper
- 2 garlic cloves, minced
- 2 tablespoons olive oil
- 4 boneless skinless chicken breast halves

Directions:

1. Heat closed contact grill for 5 minutes.
2. Meanwhile, in small bowl, combine all ingredients except chicken breast halves; mix well. Place chicken on sheet of waxed paper. Brush or rub mixture onto all sides of chicken.
3. When grill is heated, place chicken on bottom grill surface. Close grill; cook 5 to 7 minutes or until chicken is fork-tender and juices run clear.

Nutritional Information:

Serving Size: 1/4 of Recipe

Calories: 210; Calories from Fat: 100; Total Fat: 11g; Saturated Fat: 2g; Cholesterol: 75mg; Sodium: 240mg; Total Carbohydrate: 1g; Protein: 27g

2.

Oven-Roasted Potatoes and Vegetables

Ingredients:

- 2 ½ cups refrigerated new potato wedges (from 1 lb 4-oz bag)
- 1 medium red bell pepper, cut into 1-inch pieces
- 1 small zucchini, cut into 1/2-inch pieces
- 4 oz fresh whole mushrooms, quartered (about 1 cup)
- 2 teaspoons olive oil
- ½ teaspoon dried Italian seasoning
- ¼ teaspoon garlic salt

Directions:

1. Heat oven to 450°F. Spray 15x10x1-inch pan with cooking spray. In large bowl, toss all ingredients to coat. Spread evenly in pan.
2. Bake 15 to 20 minutes, stirring once halfway through baking time, until vegetables are tender and lightly browned.

Nutritional Information:

Serving Size: 2/3 Cup

Calories: 70; Calories from Fat: 15; Total Fat: 2g; Saturated Fat: 0g; Cholesterol: 0mg; Sodium: 200mg; Total Carbohydrate: 14g; Dietary Fiber: 2g; Sugars 2g ; Protein 2g

3.

Carrot Soup

Ingredients:

- 2 bags (1 lb each) ready-to-eat baby-cut carrots
- 2 large onions, chopped (about 2 cups)
- 5 ¼ cups chicken broth (from two 32-oz cartons)
- ½ teaspoon salt
- ½ cup whipping cream
- ½ cup orange juice
- 3 tablespoons packed brown sugar
- 2 tablespoons grated gingerroot
- ¼ teaspoon white pepper
- Fresh orange slices, quartered, if desired
- Fresh Italian parsley, if desired

Directions:

1. Spray 4- to 5-quart slow cooker with cooking spray. In cooker, mix carrots, onions, broth and salt.
2. Cover; cook on Low heat setting 8 to 10 hours.
3. Pour 4 cups of the soup mixture to blender; add half each of the whipping cream, orange juice, brown sugar, gingerroot and pepper. Cover and blend until smooth; return to cooker. Blend remaining soup mixture with remaining half of ingredients; return to cooker.
4. Increase heat setting to High. Cover; cook 15 to 20 minutes longer or until hot. Garnish individual servings with an orange quarter and parsley.

Nutritional Information:

Serving Size: 1 Serving

Calories: 130; Calories from Fat: 40; Total Fat: 4 1/2g; Saturated Fat: 2 1/2g; Trans Fat: 0g; Cholesterol: 15mg; Sodium: 700mg; Total Carbohydrate: 20g; Sugars: 13g; Protein: 3g.

4.

Winter Fruit Waldorf Salad

Ingredients:

- 2 medium unpeeled red apples, diced
- 2 medium unpeeled pears, diced
- ½ cup thinly sliced celery
- ½ cup golden raisins
- ½ cup chopped dates
- ¼ cup gluten-free mayonnaise or salad dressing
- ¼ cup 99% Fat Free orange crème yogurt (from 6-oz container)
- 2 tablespoons frozen orange juice concentrate
- 8 cups shredded lettuce
- Walnut halves, if desired

Directions:

1. In large bowl, mix apples, pears, celery, raisins and dates.
2. In small bowl, mix mayonnaise, yogurt and juice concentrate until well blended. Add to fruit; toss to coat. (Salad can be refrigerated up to 1 hour.) Serve on lettuce. Garnish with walnut halves.

Nutritional Information:

Serving Size: 1 Serving

Calories: 90; Calories from Fat: 25; Total Fat: 3g; Saturated Fat: 0g; Trans Fat: 0g; Cholesterol: 0mg; Sodium: 30mg; Total Carbohydrate: 16g; Dietary Fiber: 2g; Sugars: 12g; Protein: 0g.

5.

Roasted Rosemary-Onion Potatoes

Ingredients:

- 4 medium potatoes (1 1/3 pounds)
- 1 small onion, finely chopped (1/4 cup)
- 2 tablespoons olive or vegetable oil
- 2 tablespoons chopped fresh rosemary leaves or 2 teaspoons dried rosemary leaves
- 1 teaspoon chopped fresh thyme leaves or 1/4 teaspoon dried thyme leaves
- ¼ teaspoon salt
- 1/8 teaspoon pepper

Directions:

1. Heat oven to 450ºF. Grease jelly roll pan, 15 1/2x10 1/2x1 inch. Cut potatoes into 1-inch chunks.
2. Mix remaining ingredients in large bowl. Add potatoes; toss to coat. Spread potatoes in single layer in pan.
3. Bake uncovered 20 to 25 minutes, turning occasionally, until potatoes are light brown and tender when pierced with fork.

Nutritional Information:

Serving Size: 1

Calories: 185; Calories from Fat: 65; Total Fat: 7g; Saturated Fat: 1 g; Cholesterol: 0mg; Sodium: 160mg; Total Carbohydrate: 31g; Dietary Fiber: 3g; Protein: 3g

6.

Zucchini Spaghetti

Ingredients:

- 6 oz uncooked spaghetti

- 3 cups chopped zucchini (2 medium)
- 1/3 cup water
- 1 tablespoon tomato paste
- ¼ teaspoon kosher (coarse) salt
- 1/8 teaspoon coarse ground black pepper
- 1 can (15.5 oz) great northern beans, drained, rinsed
- 1 can (14.5 oz) diced tomatoes with basil, garlic and oregano, undrained
- ½ cup crumbled feta cheese (2 oz)

Directions:

1. Cook spaghetti as directed on package, omitting salt and oil; drain.
2. Meanwhile, spray 12-inch skillet with olive oil cooking spray; heat over medium-high heat. Add zucchini; cook 5 minutes, stirring occasionally, until lightly browned. Stir in water, tomato paste, salt, pepper, beans and tomatoes. Cover; simmer 4 minutes or until thoroughly heated.
3. On each of 4 plates, place about 2/3 cup spaghetti. Top each with 1 cup zucchini mixture and 2 tablespoons cheese.

Nutritional Information:

Serving Size: 1

Serving Calories 390; Total Fat: 4g; Saturated Fat: 2 1/2g; Sodium: 450 mg; Total Carbohydrate: 56g; Dietary Fiber: 7g; Protein: 34g.

7.

Chile

Ingredients:

- 2 medium unpeeled white or red potatoes (about 10 oz), cut into 1/2-inch cubes

- 1 medium onion, chopped (1/2 cup)
- 1 small bell pepper (any color), chopped (1/2 cup)
- 1 can (15 oz) chickpeas (garbanzo beans), drained, rinsed
- 1 can (15 oz) kidney beans, drained, rinsed
- 2 cans (14.5 oz each) organic diced tomatoes, undrained
- 1 can (8 oz) organic tomato sauce
- 1 tablespoon chili powder
- 1 teaspoon ground cumin
- 1 medium zucchini, cut into 1/2-inch slices

Directions:

1. In 4-quart Dutch oven, place all ingredients except zucchini; stir well. Heat to boiling over high heat, stirring occasionally; reduce heat. Cover; simmer 10 minutes.
2. Stir in zucchini. Cover; cook 5 to 7 minutes longer, stirring occasionally, until potatoes and zucchini are tender when pierced with fork.

Nutritional Information:

Serving Size: 1

Serving Calories: 280; Calories from Fat: 25; Total Fat: 2 1/2g; Saturated Fat: 0g;Trans Fat: 0g; Cholesterol: 0mg; Sodium: 650 mg; Total Carbohydrate: 51g; Dietary Fiber: 12g; Sugars: 8g; Protein: 4g.

8.

Herb & Garlic Chicken with Vegetables

Ingredients:

- 1 cut-up whole chicken (3 to 3 1/2 lb)
- 2 tablespoons olive or vegetable oil
- 1 envelope savory herb with garlic soup mix (from 2.4-oz box)
- 1/3 cup chicken broth

- 4 medium stalks celery, cut in half lengthwise, then cut into 4-inch pieces
- 1 large onion, cut into 6 wedges
- 2 large carrots, cut in half lengthwise, then cut into 4-inch pieces
- 2 medium unpeeled russet potatoes, each cut into 8 pieces

Directions:

1. Heat oven to 425°F. Remove skin from chicken if desired. In small bowl, mix oil, soup mix and broth. Brush both sides of chicken pieces with about half of the oil mixture.
2. In large bowl, mix celery, onion, carrots, potatoes and remaining oil mixture. Arrange vegetables in ungreased 15x10x1-inch pan. Bake 15 minutes.
3. Place chicken pieces in pan, overlapping vegetables if necessary. Bake 35 to 40 minutes longer or until vegetables are tender and juice of chicken is clear when thickest piece is cut to bone (170°F for breasts; 180°F for thighs and legs).

Nutritional Information:

Serving Size: 1

Serving Calories: 450; Calories from Fat: 150; Total Fat 17g;Saturated Fat 3 1/2g; Trans Fat 0g; Cholesterol 120mg; Sodium:990mg; Total Carbohydrate: 32g; Dietary Fiber: 5g; Sugars: 6g; Protein: 42g.

9.

Roasted Salmon and Vegetables

Ingredients:

- 4 salmon steaks, ½ inch thick (about 1 ½ lb)
- 2 cups refrigerated new potato wedges with skins (from 20-oz bag)

- 2 small zucchini, quartered lengthwise, then cut into 2-inch pieces
- 1 medium red bell pepper, cut into 2-inch pieces
- 1 tablespoon lemon juice
- 1 tablespoon butter or margarine, melted
- ½ teaspoon salt
- ¼ to ½ teaspoon dried tarragon leaves
- ¼ teaspoon pepper

Directions:

1. Heat oven to 425°F. Place salmon steaks in ungreased 15x10x1-inch pan. Arrange potato wedges, zucchini and bell pepper around salmon.
2. Brush salmon with lemon juice. Brush salmon and vegetables with butter; sprinkle with salt, tarragon and pepper.
3. Bake 25 to 35 minutes or until salmon flakes easily with fork and vegetables are tender.

Nutritional Information:

Serving Size: 1 Serving

Calories: 290; Calories from Fat: 100; Total Fat: 11g; Saturated Fat: 4g; Trans Fat: 0g; Cholesterol: 105mg; Sodium 490: mg; Total Carbohydrate 14g; Dietary Fiber: 3g; Sugars: 4g; Protein: 34g.

10.

Banana-Blueberry Smoothie

Ingredients:

- 1 cup milk
- 1 cup Cheerios cereal

- 1 ripe banana, cut into chunks
- 1 cup fresh blueberries
- 1 cup ice
- Garnishes, If Desired
- Banana slices
- Additional cereal

Directions:

1. In blender, place Smoothie ingredients. Cover; blend on high speed about 30 seconds or until smooth.
2. Pour into 2 glasses. Garnish as desired. Serve immediately.

Serving Size: 1 Serving

Calories: 240; Calories from Fat: 35; Total Fat 4g; Saturated Fat: 2g; Trans Fat: 0g; Cholesterol 10mg; Sodium: 170mg; Total Carbohydrate: 45g; Dietary Fiber: 4g; Sugars: 27g; Protein: 6g.

11.

Cherry Strawberry Smoothie

Ingredients:

- 2 containers (5.3 oz each) honey Greek yogurt
- 1 ½ cups frozen organic cherries
- ½ cup frozen organic strawberries
- 1 cup milk

Directions:

1. In blender, place all ingredients. Cover and blend on high speed about 1 minute or until smooth.
2. Pour into 3 glasses. Serve immediately.

Serving Size: 1 Serving

Calories: 230; Calories from Fat: 30; Total Fat: 3 1/2g; Saturated Fat: 2g; Trans Fat: 0g; Cholesterol: 5mg; Sodium: 65mg; Total Carbohydrate: 38g; Dietary Fiber: 2g; Sugars: 34g; Protein: 11g;

12.

Berry Breakfast Quinoa

Ingredients:

- ¼ cup milk
- 2 containers (6 oz each) 99% Fat Free French vanilla, strawberry or peach yogurt
- 4 teaspoons chia seed
- 1 cup cooled cooked quinoa (1/4 cup uncooked)
- 2 cups fresh fruit (mixed berries or chopped peaches)
- ¼ cup coarsely chopped toasted almonds or pecans
- 1/8 teaspoon ground cinnamon

Directions:

1. In medium bowl, stir together milk, yogurt and chia seed until blended. Evenly divide mixture among 4 glasses. Spoon 1/4 cup cooled cooked quinoa on top of yogurt layer on each.
2. Top each with a layer of fruit and almonds. Sprinkle with cinnamon. Let stand 5 minutes, or cover and refrigerate overnight.

Serving Size: 1

Serving Calories: 260; Calories from Fat: 70 Total Fat8g;   Saturated Fat: 1 1/2g; Trans Fat 0g; Cholesterol 5mg; Sodium: 80mg; Total Carbohydrate: 40g; Dietary Fiber: 4g; Sugars: 24g; Protein: 8g.

13.

Quinoa and Vegetable Salad

Ingredients:

- 1 cup uncooked quinoa
- 2 tablespoons fresh lemon juice
- 2 tablespoons olive oil
- 2 tablespoons chopped fresh basil
- 1 can (15 oz) gluten-free garbanzo beans, drained, rinsed
- 1 can (15.25 oz) gluten-free whole kernel sweet corn, drained
- 1 can (14.5 oz) gluten-free diced tomatoes, drained
- 1 cup chopped red bell pepper
- 1/3 cup quartered pitted olives
- ½ cup crumbled gluten-free feta cheese

Directions:

1. Rinse quinoa under cold water 1 minute; drain. Cook quinoa as directed on package; drain. Cool completely, about 30 minutes.
2. Meanwhile, in small nonmetal bowl, place lemon juice, oil and basil; mix well. Set aside for dressing.
3. In large bowl, gently toss cooked quinoa, beans, corn, tomatoes, bell pepper and olives. Pour dressing over quinoa mixture; toss gently to coat. Serve immediately or refrigerate 1 to 2 hours before serving.
4. Just before serving, sprinkle with cheese. Garnish with basil leaves if desired.

Nutritional Information:

Serving Size: 1 Serving

Calories: 350; Calories from Fat: 100; Total Fat: 12g; Saturated Fat: 3g; Trans Fat: 0g; Cholesterol 10mg; Sodium: 580mg; Total Carbohydrate: 49g; Dietary Fiber: 7g; Sugars: 7g; Protein: 12.

14.

Creamy Fruit Tarts

Ingredients:

- 1 cup Bisquick mix
- 2 tablespoons sugar
- 1 tablespoon butter or margarine, softened
- 2 packages (3 ounces each) cream cheese, softened
- ¼ cup sugar
- ¼ cup sour cream
- 1 ½ cups assorted sliced fresh fruit or berries
- 1/3 cup apple jelly, melted

Directions:

1. Heat oven to 375°F. Mix Bisquick, 2 tablespoons sugar, the butter and 1 package cream cheese in small bowl until dough forms a ball.
2. Divide dough into 6 parts. Press each part dough on bottom and 3/4 inch up side in each of 6 tart pans, 4 1/4 x 1 inch, or 10-ounce custard cups. Place on cookie sheet.
3. Bake 10 to 12 minutes or until light brown. Cool in pans on wire rack, about 30 minutes. Remove tart shells from pans.
4. Beat remaining package cream cheese, 1/4 cup sugar and the sour cream until smooth. Spoon into tart shells, spreading over bottoms. Top each with about 1/4 cup fruit. Brush with jelly.

Nutritional Information:

Serving Size: 1 Serving

Calories: 320; Calories from Fat: 155; Total Fat 17g; Saturated Fat;
8g; Cholesterol: 35mg; Sodium: 400mg; Total Carbohydrate: 40g;
Dietary Fiber: 2 g; Protein 4g.

Chapter 8: The Wrap

I had a lot of goals when I set out to write this book, but the most important of these was to shed light on the gout and how to beat it.

You have one life to live. If you have gout, it is not a death sentence, but rather, a wake-up call for you to take better care of yourself. Think of it as a blessing in disguise. You are going to have to make some changes. That's it.

Whether you need to take medicine for it or not you should ensure that you follow these simple rules of thumb:

- Limit alcoholic beverages and drinks sweetened with fruit sugar (fructose).
- Drink plenty of nonalcoholic beverages, especially water.
- Limit intake of foods high in purines, such as red meat, organ meats and seafood.
- Exercise regularly and lose weight. Keeping your body at a healthy weight reduces your risk of gout.

I hope you enjoyed this book and found it useful.   Now that you have a basic understanding of gout and its causes and remedies, I want you to act on what you have learned and BEAT gout into your past, where it belongs.

.

Glossary

Acute gout: An acute condition which is caused by a disorder of purine or pyrimidine metabolism resulting in inflammatory arthritis.

Allopurinol : One of the oldest medications used to treat gout. Allopurinol works by preventing uric acid production.

Ankle conditions: Conditions that affect the ankle.

Arthritis: General name for any type of joint inflammation, but often means age-related osteoarthritis.

Arthritis-like conditions: Medical conditions highly related to or similar to arthritis.

Asymptomatic hyperuricemia: The term applied to settings in which the serum urate concentration is elevated but in which neither symptoms nor signs of urate crystal deposition (gout) have occurred.

Big toe swelling: Edema or swelling of the big toe.

Bursitis: Inflammation of one or more bursae (small sacs) of synovial fluid in the body.

Cellulitis: Inflammation of skin or subcutaneous tissues.

Chemical poisoning -- Molybdenum: Molybdenum is a chemical used mainly in steel alloys lubricants. Ingestion and other exposures to the chemical can cause various symptoms. The type and severity of symptoms varies depending on the amount of chemical involved and the nature of the exposure.

Colchicine - Colchicine is a medication prescribed to reduce inflammation associated with gout. Grapefruit or grapefruit juice should not be consumed when taking Colchicine.

Chronic gout: Repeated episodes of pain and inflammation. More than one joint may be affected. Gout is caused by having higher-than-normal levels of uric acid in your body.

Chronic kidney failure: Gradual failure of the kidneys over a period of time.

Crystal deposit disease: A group of diseases characterized by the deposit of crystals in body tissues. Some examples of such disorders includes scleroderma, dermatomyositis, arthritis and kidney disease. The severity and type of symptoms depend on the nature and location of the crystals deposited.

Fatigue: Excessive tiredness or weakness.

Glycogen Storage Disease Type I: An inherited metabolic disorder where a deficiency of the enzyme glucose-6-phosphatase prevents glycogen being turned into glucose leading to a buildup of glycogen in the liver and kidneys. Most problems tend to develop during adulthood.

Glycogen storage disease type 7: An inherited metabolic disorder where there is a deficiency of phosphofructokinase-1 in the muscle and a partial deficiency in red blood cells which prevents glucose being converted to energy during exercise.

Gout : Historically known as "the disease of kings" or "rich man's disease" - gout is an acute and extremely painful form of arthritis which can affect a number of joints in the body, including the ankle, the wrist, the knee and the elbow , but most commonly begins in the joint of the big toe.

Hereditary gout: Gout that runs in families.

Hyperuricemia : High blood levels of uric acid.

Joint pain: Pain affecting the joints.

Juvenile gout: Gout that occurs in children as a result of kidney disease caused by a genetic defect.

Kidney damage: Any damage that occurs to the kidneys.

Kidney stones: Kidney stones are solid deposits of salts (e.g calcium) from the urine. These deposits can impair the passage of urine that has the potential to result in infection and kidney damage or failure in severe cases.

Knee conditions: Any condition that affects the knee.

Lead poisoning: A type of heavy metal poisoning caused by excessive exposure to lead.

Limb conditions: Medical conditions affecting the upper or lower limbs.

Medullary cystic kidney disease 2: A rare disorder characterized mainly by the development of kidney cysts and affects kidney function during adulthood. The disorder is caused by a genetic defect (chromosome 16p12.3). Type 2 tends to have an earlier onset of end stage kidney failure.

Metatarsal-phalangeal joint - the joint at the base of the big toe is the most commonly affected with approximately 50% of cases.

Muscle phosphoglycerate kinase deficiency: An inherited genetic muscle disease where an enzyme deficiency (phosphoglycerate kinase) affects the normal processes that convert carbohydrates from food into energy.

Musculoskeletal conditions: Medical conditions affecting the musculoskeletal system of bones, muscles and related structures.

No symptoms: The absence of noticeable symptoms.

Non-pathogenic inflammatory conditions: Medical disorders that cause inflammation, but are not due to any infectious pathogen.

Osteoarthritis: Osteoarthritis is a chronic condition characterized by mechanical disturbances due to degradation of joints. It is the most common form of arthritis, and the leading cause of chronic disability.

Pain conditions: Diseases characterized by pain and pain-like symptoms.

Palindromic rheumatism: A rare disorder involving periodic inflammation in and around joints. Eventually, rheumatoid arthritis may develop if the condition persists.

Podagra: A condition which is characterized by a gout like pain in the toe.

Poly-articular Gout: A form of arthritic condition that is the result of painful crystals forming in the joints. These crystals form due to increased amounts of uric acid in your blood.

Pseudo-gout: The symptoms of gout often mimic those of pseudo-gout, or "false gout". The difference is between the two is that while gout is characterized by uric acid crystals; pseudo-gout is characterized by calcium in the joint, especially in the knee.

Psoriatic Arthritis: Psoriatic arthritis is a chronic disease characterized by inflammation of the skin (psoriasis) and joints (arthritis). Psoriatic arthritis is said to be a seronegative spondyloarthropathy and therefore occurs more commonly in patients with tissue type HLA-B27.

Purines: Purines are a compound found in some food sources. During the process of digestion, purine-rich foods such as red meat and seafood release uric acid into the blood. Elevated uric acid levels contribute to the development of gout.

Reactive arthritis: The inflammation of a joint.

Rheumatic conditions: Any condition that affects ones joints.

Stiff joints: Reduced mobility or movement of the joints.

Stress: Emotional stress (sometimes refers to physical stress).

Surgical errors/complications: Any error or complication that arises from surgery.

Toe pain: Pain affecting one or more toes.

Tophi - Tophi are uric acid crystals that accumulate in the soft tissue of the joint. Tophi often form in the elbow, fingers or toes and can cause joint damage. Tophi can also form in the ears.

Uric acid - Uric acid is a by-product of purine digestion. Blood uric acid levels are often elevated in individuals with gout. The aim of gout treatment is to lower uric acid levels through changes to diet, weight loss or via medications.

Uric acid crystals - Uric acid crystals may form in joints in the presence of excess uric acid. These crystals are identified as foreign invaders and 'attacked' by the immune system. This attack results in intense pain, swelling and inflammation (often experienced as a sharp and/or burning sensations).

Urinary stones: Stones in the urinary tract or bladder.

Urate: A salt derived from uric acid. When the body cannot metabolize uric acid properly, urates can build up in body tissues or crystallize within the joints.

Von Gierke Disease: An inherited metabolic disorder where a deficiency of the enzyme glucose-6-phosphatase prevents glycogen being turned into glucose leading to a buildup of glycogen in the liver and kidneys.

www.ingramcontent.com/pod-product-compliance
Lightning Source LLC
Chambersburg PA
CBHW072120280526
45788CB00006B/2574